Mediterranean High Blood Pressure

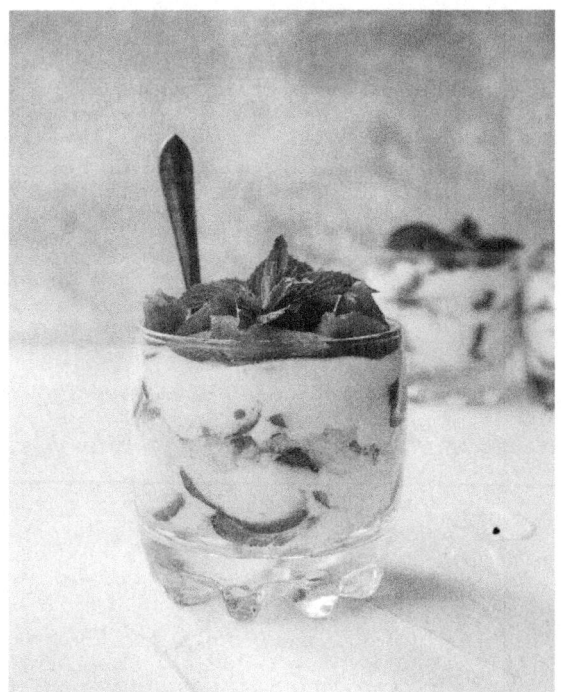

Delicious Quick and easy 30 Recipes to improve your health and feel great

Copyright © 2023 by Zeerah Amelia

All rights reserved. No part of this book may be reproduced, stored in a retrieval system, or transmitted in any form or by any means, electronic, mechanical, photocopying, recording, or otherwise, without prior written permission from the publisher.

Disclaimer Notice: Please note the information contained within this document is for educational and entertainment purposes only. Under no circumstances will any blame or legal responsibility be held against the publisher, or author, for any damages, reparation, or monetary loss due to the information contained within this book, either directly or indirectly.

All effort has been executed to present accurate, up-to-date, reliable, and complete information. No warranties of any kind are declared or implied.

NOTICE: For your safety and that of others, especially Children, be careful using Sharp knives, glass, hot pans and heated cooking surfaces while working with these recipes. Keep children at a safe distance from the stove during the cooking process and while leaving food to cool.

TABLE OF CONTENTS

INTRODUCTION 5

Understanding High Blood Pressure 6

Healthy and Delicious Recipes to Manage and Prevent High Blood Pressure 8

Breakfast Recipes: 9
   1. Greek Yogurt Parfait 9
   2. Avocado Toast 10
   3. Mediterranean Omelette 12
   4. Mediterranean Breakfast Smoothie 14
   5. Simple Fruit Salad 15

Lunch Recipes: 17
   6. Greek Chickpea Salad 17
   7. Mediterranean Stuffed Peppers 19
   8. Mediterranean Tuna Salad 20
   9. Mediterranean Hummus Wrap 22
   10. Mediterranean Lentil Soup 23

Dinner Recipes 25
   11. Mediterranean Baked Salmon 25
   12. Mediterranean Quinoa Salad 27
   12. Mediterranean Grilled Chicken 29

14. Mediterranean Roasted Vegetables 30
15. Mediterranean Shrimp Stir-Fry 32
Snacks Recipes 34
16. Mediterranean Hummus Dip 34
17. Greek Yogurt and Cucumber Dip 35
18. Mediterranean Stuffed Grape Leaves 37
19. Mediterranean Tomato Bruschetta 39
20. Mediterranean Stuffed Mushrooms 40
Desserts Recipes 42
21. Mediterranean Fresh Fruit Salad 42
22. Greek Yogurt with Honey and Walnuts 44
23. Mediterranean Orange and Almond Cake 45
24. Mediterranean Yogurt Parfait with Berries and Pistachios 47
25. Mediterranean Chocolate-Dipped Figs 49
Smoothies Recipes 50
26. Mediterranean Green Smoothie 50
27. Mediterranean Berry Smoothie 52
28. Mediterranean Tropical Smoothie 53
29. Mediterranean Avocado Banana Smoothie 55
30. Mediterranean Chia Seed Pudding Smoothie 57
CONCLUSION 59

INTRODUCTION

Are you tired of battling constantly with high blood pressure and struggling to find the right diet? What if I told you that there is a delicious way to take charge of your health and lower your blood pressure? Imagine a life where you can savor delectable dishes while effortlessly managing your hypertension. That life is within your reach, and I can attest to it firsthand.

I'm Zeerah, and I was once grappling with the challenges of high blood pressure. Frustrated and seeking answers, I embarked on a quest to find a solution. Extensive research and guidance from health experts led me to discover the power of the Mediterranean diet in managing hypertension.

By embracing the wholesome goodness of this diet and incorporating heart-healthy foods into my daily meals, my blood pressure stabilized, and my overall well-being improved. Motivated by my own transformation, I felt compelled to share my knowledge and experience with others facing a similar battle.

That's why I've crafted this book, "Delicious Mediterranean Diet for High Blood Pressure: Embrace Flavorful Foods for Better Health." It's a comprehensive resource that equips you with all the tools and information you need to take control of your blood pressure.

Within these pages, you'll find carefully curated recipes that serve as your go-to guide when planning meals and making healthier choices. Additionally, I've included 30 delightful and nutritious recipes that not only support your heart health but also tickle your taste buds.

I invite you to join me on this transformative journey towards better health. Together, let's discover the joys of the Mediterranean diet and regain control over our blood pressure. Let this book be your roadmap to a life of vitality and freedom from the burdens of hypertension. Take the first step today and embrace this delicious and heart-healthy diet that will positively change your life forever.

Understanding High Blood Pressure

The Mediterranean diet is a delightful and effective way to shed those extra pounds and take control of your high blood pressure. It's not just a diet; it's a lifestyle that centers around fresh and wholesome foods inspired by the traditional eating habits of Mediterranean countries like Greece and Italy.

Imagine savoring a colorful plate of succulent tomatoes, crisp cucumbers, and creamy feta cheese drizzled with olive oil, all topped off with a sprinkling of aromatic herbs. That's just a glimpse of the vibrant flavors this diet offers! The Mediterranean diet emphasizes vegetables, fruits, whole grains, nuts, and legumes, providing a rich array of nutrients to nourish your body.

What's truly remarkable is the Mediterranean diet's ability to support weight loss and tackle high blood pressure. By swapping out unhealthy fats with heart-healthy olive oil, you're reducing your risk of heart disease and aiding in weight management. Plus, the abundance of fiber keeps you feeling full and satisfied, curbing those pesky cravings.

This diet also promotes moderate consumption of lean proteins, like fish and poultry, while minimizing red meat. These choices help maintain a healthy weight and lower blood pressure, reducing strain on the cardiovascular system.

Additionally, the Mediterranean diet encourages enjoying meals with family and friends, fostering a positive relationship with food and reducing stress—a major factor in hypertension.

Incorporating the Mediterranean diet into your life can be a transformative journey, not just for your weight and blood pressure but also for your overall well-being. Remember, it's not a rigid plan; it's about relishing the delicious flavors, savoring the moments shared around the table, and embracing a lifestyle that nurtures your body and mind.

Healthy and Delicious Recipes to Manage and Prevent High Blood Pressure

Embark on a Flavorful Journey: Mediterranean Diet for Weight Loss and Lowering High Blood Pressure

Embrace a vibrant and satisfying approach to manage high blood pressure and achieve weight loss without compromising on taste. Our vast collection of mouthwatering Mediterranean diet recipes ensures you relish quick, wholesome, and delightful meals, ideal for breakfast, lunch, dinner, snacks, desserts, and smoothies. These thoughtfully crafted recipes are your ticket to controlling high blood pressure while savoring every flavorful dish. Begin your journey today!"

Breakfast Recipes:

1. *Greek Yogurt Parfait*

Prep Time: 5 minutes

Serving: 1

Ingredients:

- 1 cup Greek yogurt
- 1/2 cup mixed berries (blueberries, strawberries, raspberries)
- 2 tablespoons honey
- 2 tablespoons granola

Directions:

- Greek yogurt, mixed berries, and honey should be layered in a glass.
- Top with some granola.
- Serve right away.

Nutrition Info:

- Calories: 350
- Carbs: 45g
- Protein: 18g
- Fat: 10g

- Fiber: 5g

Grocery Shopping List:

- Greek yogurt
- Mixed berries (fresh or frozen)
- Honey
- Granola

Frequent Q&A:

Can I use regular yogurt instead of Greek yogurt? Yes, you can, but Greek yogurt has more protein.

Can I add nuts to the parfait? Absolutely, it will add extra crunch and healthy fats.

Utensils:

- Glass for serving

2. *Avocado Toast*

Prep Time: 5 minutes

Serving: 1

Ingredients:

- 1 ripe avocado
- 2 slices whole-grain bread

- 1 teaspoon lemon juice
- Pinch of salt and pepper

Directions:

- In a bowl, mash the avocado and stir in the lemon juice, salt, and pepper.
- Bread pieces should be toasted till golden brown.
- On the bread, equally distribute the mashed avocado.
- Serve right away.

Nutrition Info:

- Calories: 300
- Carbs: 30g
- Protein: 8g
- Fat: 18g
- Fiber: 10g

Grocery Shopping List:

- Avocado
- Whole-grain bread
- Lemon
- Salt and pepper

Frequent Q&A:

Can I add a poached egg on top? Yes, a poached egg can add extra protein and flavor.

Can I use any bread? Yes, but choose whole-grain or whole-wheat for added nutrition.

Utensils:

Bowl for mashing avocado

Toaster

3. *Mediterranean Omelette*

Prep Time: 5 minutes

Serving: 1

Ingredients:

- 3 eggs
- 1/4 cup cherry tomatoes, halved
- 2 tablespoons feta cheese, crumbled
- 1 tablespoon fresh parsley, chopped

Directions:

- In a bowl, whisk the eggs until well mixed.
- Over medium heat, pour the beaten eggs into a nonstick pan.
- On one side of the omelette, sprinkle feta cheese and cherry tomatoes.
- When the cheese has melted, fold the omelette in half and cook for one more minute.

- Serve after adding fresh parsley as a garnish.

Nutrition Info:

- Calories: 350
- Carbs: 5g
- Protein: 23g
- Fat: 26g
- Fiber: 1g

Grocery Shopping List:

- Eggs
- Cherry tomatoes
- Feta cheese
- Fresh parsley

Frequent Q&A:

Can I add spinach or other veggies? Absolutely, feel free to customize with your favorite vegetables.

Can I use other cheeses? Yes, goat cheese or mozzarella would work well too.

Utensils:

- Bowl for beating eggs
- Non-stick pan

4. Mediterranean Breakfast Smoothie

Prep Time: 5 minutes

Serving: 1

Ingredients:

- 1/2 cup Greek yogurt
- 1/2 cup unsweetened almond milk
- 1/2 cup frozen mixed berries (blueberries, strawberries, raspberries)
- 1 tablespoon chia seeds

Directions:

- Greek yogurt, almond milk, and frozen berries should all be put in a blender.
- Blend till creamy and smooth.
- Add chia seeds after pouring into a glass.
- Serve right away.

Nutrition Info:

- Calories: 250
- Carbs: 25g
- Protein: 15g
- Fat: 10g
- Fiber: 10g

Grocery Shopping List:

- Greek yogurt
- Unsweetened almond milk
- Frozen mixed berries
- Chia seeds

Frequent Q&A:

Can I use regular milk instead of almond milk? Yes, any milk will work fine.

Can I add a banana for sweetness? Absolutely, bananas will add natural sweetness.

Utensils:

Blender

5. Simple Fruit Salad

Prep Time: 5 minutes

Serving: 1

Ingredients:

- 1 cup mixed fruits (apple, orange, grapes, melon)
- 1 tablespoon fresh lemon juice
- 1 teaspoon honey

Directions:

- Fruits should be washed and cut into bite-sized pieces.
- Fruits, lemon juice, and honey should all be combined in one bowl.
- Gently toss the fruits until they are evenly covered with the dressing.
- Serve right away.

Nutrition Info:

- Calories: 150
- Carbs: 35g
- Protein: 1g
- Fat: 0g
- Fiber: 5g

Grocery Shopping List:

- Mixed fruits (apple, orange, grapes, melon)
- Lemon
- Honey

Frequent Q&A:

Can I add mint leaves for extra freshness? Absolutely, mint leaves would be a great addition.

Can I use canned fruits? Fresh fruits are recommended for maximum nutritional benefits.

Utensils:

Bowl for mixing fruits

Fork for tossing

Lunch Recipes:

6. Greek Chickpea Salad

Prep Time: 10 minutes

Serving: 2

Ingredients:

- 1 can chickpeas, drained and rinsed
- 1 cucumber, diced
- 1 cup cherry tomatoes, halved
- 1/2 red onion, thinly sliced

Directions:

- Chickpeas, cucumber, cherry tomatoes, and red onion should all be combined in a big bowl.
- To equally combine the ingredients, gently toss.
- Use your preferred Mediterranean dressing or a concoction of olive oil, lemon juice, and herbs as a drizzle.
- Serve Chilled

Nutrition Info:

- Calories: 250
- Carbs: 40g
- Protein: 12g
- Fat: 4g
- Fiber: 10g

Grocery Shopping List:

- Chickpeas (canned or dried)
- Cucumber
- Cherry tomatoes
- Red onion
- Mediterranean dressing or olive oil, lemon juice, and herbs

Frequent Q&A:

Can I add olives and feta cheese? Yes, they will enhance the Mediterranean flavors.

Can I make this salad ahead of time? Yes, it will keep well in the refrigerator for a day.

Utensils:

Large bowl for mixing

7. Mediterranean Stuffed Peppers

Prep Time: 15 minutes

Serving: 2

Ingredients:

- 2 large bell peppers (red, yellow, or orange)
- 1 cup cooked quinoa or couscous
- 1/2 cup canned chickpeas, drained and rinsed
- 1/2 cup diced tomatoes (canned or fresh)

Directions:

- Set the oven's temperature to 375°F (190°C).
- Bell peppers should have the tops cut off and the seeds taken out.
- Chickpeas, chopped tomatoes, and cooked quinoa or couscous should be combined in a dish.
- Fill the bell peppers with the mixture.
- The filled peppers should be baked for 20 to 25 minutes, or until they are soft.
- Serve warm.

Nutrition Info:

- Calories: 300
- Carbs: 60g
- Protein: 10g
- Fat: 2g

- Fiber: 10g

Grocery Shopping List:

- Bell peppers
- Quinoa or couscous
- Canned chickpeas
- Diced tomatoes (canned or fresh)

Frequent Q&A:

Can I add spinach or other veggies to the stuffing? Yes, feel free to add your favorite vegetables.

Can I use other grains instead of quinoa or couscous? Yes, brown rice or bulgur will work well too.

Utensils:

Baking dish

8. Mediterranean Tuna Salad

Prep Time: 10 minutes

Serving: 1

Ingredients:

- 1 can tuna, drained
- 1/4 cup chopped cucumber
- 1/4 cup chopped red bell pepper

- 1 tablespoon olive oil

Directions:

- Tuna, sliced cucumber, and red bell pepper should all be combined in a bowl.
- Add a drizzle of olive oil and blend gently.
- To taste, add salt and pepper to the food.
- Serve as a sandwich filler or over a bed of mixed greens.

Nutrition Info:

- Calories: 250
- Carbs: 5g
- Protein: 25g
- Fat: 16g
- Fiber: 1g

Grocery Shopping List:

- Canned tuna
- Cucumber
- Red bell pepper
- Olive oil

Frequent Q&A:

Can I add olives or capers for extra flavor? Yes, they will complement the tuna salad nicely.

Can I use canned salmon instead of tuna? Yes, canned salmon works well too.

Utensils:

Bowl for mixing

9. *Mediterranean Hummus Wrap*

Prep Time: 10 minutes

Serving: 1

Ingredients:

- 1 whole-grain tortilla
- 1/2 cup hummus
- 1/4 cup shredded carrots
- 1/4 cup sliced cucumber

Directions:

- The whole-grain tortilla should be placed level on a tidy surface.
- Over the tortilla, evenly distribute the hummus.
- Sliced cucumber and carrots should be added on top.
- To make a wrap, firmly roll the tortilla.
- Slice in half, then serve.

Nutrition Info:

- Calories: 350
- Carbs: 45g
- Protein: 10g

- Fat: 15g
- Fiber: 8g

Grocery Shopping List:

- Whole-grain tortilla
- Hummus
- Carrots
- Cucumber

Frequent Q&A:

Can I add grilled chicken for extra protein? Yes, grilled chicken is a great addition.

Can I use other types of hummus? Yes, roasted red pepper or black bean hummus would be delicious too.

Utensils:

Cutting board and knife

10. Mediterranean Lentil Soup

Prep Time: 15 minutes

Serving: 4

Ingredients:

- 1 cup dried lentils
- 1/2 cup diced onion

- 1/2 cup diced carrots
- 1/2 cup diced tomatoes (canned or fresh)

Directions:

- Drain the lentils after giving them a cold water rinse.
- Diced onion and carrots should be sautéed in a big saucepan until they soften.
- Add lentils and diced tomatoes to the pot.
- Fill the lentils up with water or vegetable broth.
- When the lentils are ready, simmer for about 20 minutes after bringing to a boil.
- To taste, add salt and pepper to the food.
- Serve warm.

Nutrition Info:

- Calories: 200
- Carbs: 30g
- Protein: 15g
- Fat: 1g
- Fiber: 15g

Grocery Shopping List:

- Dried lentils
- Onion
- Carrots
- Diced tomatoes (canned or fresh)
- Vegetable broth

Frequent Q&A:

Can I add spinach or kale for extra greens? Yes, they will enhance the nutritional value.

Can I make this soup in a slow cooker? Absolutely, just adjust the cooking time accordingly.

Utensils:

Large pot for cooking

Dinner Recipes

11. Mediterranean Baked Salmon

Prep Time: 10 minutes

Serving: 2

Ingredients:

- 2 salmon fillets
- 1 lemon, sliced
- 2 cloves garlic, minced
- 1 tablespoon olive oil

Directions:

- Preheat the oven to 375°F (190°C).

- Place the salmon fillets on a baking sheet lined with parchment paper.
- Drizzle olive oil over the salmon and rub minced garlic on top.
- Arrange lemon slices on the salmon.
- Bake for 15-20 minutes or until the salmon is cooked through.
- Serve hot.

Nutrition Info:

- Calories: 400
- Carbs: 2g
- Protein: 30g
- Fat: 30g
- Fiber: 1g

Grocery Shopping List:

- Salmon fillets
- Lemon
- Garlic
- Olive oil

Frequent Q&A:

Can I add herbs like dill or parsley for extra flavor? Yes, fresh herbs will enhance the taste.

Can I grill the salmon instead of baking? Yes, grilling is another tasty option.

Utensils:

Baking sheet and parchment paper

12. Mediterranean Quinoa Salad

Prep Time: 15 minutes

Serving: 2

Ingredients:

- 1 cup cooked quinoa
- 1/2 cup chopped cucumber
- 1/2 cup chopped tomatoes
- 1/4 cup crumbled feta cheese

Directions:

- Cucumber, tomatoes, and cooked quinoa should all be combined in a dish.
- Feta cheese crumbles should be added on top.
- Toss everything together carefully.
- Drizzle with your preferred olive oil and lemon juice or Mediterranean dressing.
- Serve Chilled.

Nutrition Info:

- Calories: 300
- Carbs: 40g
- Protein: 10g
- Fat: 12g
- Fiber: 5g

Grocery Shopping List:

- Quinoa
- Cucumber
- Tomatoes
- Feta cheese
- Mediterranean dressing or olive oil, lemon juice

Frequent Q&A:

Can I add olives or artichoke hearts? Yes, they will add extra Mediterranean flavors.

Can I use couscous instead of quinoa? Yes, couscous is a great alternative.

Utensils:

Bowl for mixing

12. Mediterranean Grilled Chicken

Prep Time: 10 minutes

Serving: 2

Ingredients:

- 2 chicken breasts
- 1 tablespoon olive oil
- 1 tablespoon lemon juice
- 1 teaspoon dried oregano

Directions:

- To prepare a marinade, combine olive oil, lemon juice, and dried oregano in a basin.
- As you add the chicken breasts to the marinade, make sure to thoroughly coat them.
- Refrigerate for at least 30 minutes with a cover on.
- A grill or grill pan should be preheated to high heat.
- The chicken breasts should be cooked through after grilling for 5 to 6 minutes on each side.
- Serve warm.

Nutrition Info:

- Calories: 300
- Carbs: 1g
- Protein: 40g
- Fat: 14g

- Fiber: 0g

Grocery Shopping List:

- Chicken breasts
- Olive oil
- Lemon
- Dried oregano

Frequent Q&A:

Can I add garlic to the marinade? Absolutely, minced garlic will add extra flavor.

Can I use boneless chicken thighs instead of breasts? Yes, boneless chicken thighs will work well too.

Utensils:

Grill or grill pan

14. Mediterranean Roasted Vegetables

Prep Time: 10 minutes

Serving: 2

Ingredients:

- 2 cups mixed vegetables (zucchini, bell peppers, eggplant)
- 1 tablespoon olive oil

- 1 teaspoon dried thyme

Directions:

- Set the oven's temperature to 425°F (220°C).
- Bite-sized portions of the mixed veggies should be used.
- Olive oil and dried thyme should be combined with the veggies in a dish.
- On a baking sheet covered with parchment paper, spread out the veggies.
- Vegetables should be roasted for 15 to 20 minutes, or until they are soft and slightly browned.
- Serve warm.

Nutrition Info:

- Calories: 200
- Carbs: 20g
- Protein: 5g
- Fat: 10g
- Fiber: 10g

Grocery Shopping List:

- Zucchini
- Bell peppers
- Eggplant
- Olive oil
- Dried thyme

Frequent Q&A:

Can I add balsamic vinegar for extra tanginess? Yes, a drizzle of balsamic vinegar will enhance the flavors.

Can I use other vegetables? Yes, any vegetables you enjoy will work well in this recipe.

Utensils:

Baking sheet and parchment paper

15. Mediterranean Shrimp Stir-Fry

Prep Time: 15 minutes

Serving: 2

Ingredients:

- 1-pound shrimp, peeled and deveined
- 1 cup sliced bell peppers (assorted colors)
- 1 cup sliced zucchini
- 2 tablespoons olive oil

Directions:

- Olive oil should be heated to a medium-high haze in a big skillet.
- When the shrimp are pink and cooked through, add them to the skillet and cook for 2-3 minutes on each side.

- Sliced bell peppers and zucchini should be added to the skillet.
- Once the veggies are tender-crisp, stir-fry for a further 2-3 minutes.
- To taste, add salt and pepper to the food.
- Serve warm.

Nutrition Info:

- Calories: 250
- Carbs: 8g
- Protein: 30g
- Fat: 12g
- Fiber: 3g

Grocery Shopping List:

- Shrimp
- Bell peppers
- Zucchini
- Olive oil

Frequent Q&A:

Can I add garlic and lemon for extra flavor? Yes, they will enhance the taste of the dish.

Can I use chicken instead of shrimp? Yes, sliced chicken breast would be a good alternative.

Utensils:

Large skillet

Snacks Recipes

16. Mediterranean Hummus Dip

Prep Time: 5 minutes

Serving: 4

Ingredients:

- 1 can chickpeas, drained and rinsed
- 1/4 cup tahini
- 1/4 cup lemon juice
- 2 cloves garlic, minced

Directions:

- Combine the chickpeas, tahini, lemon juice, and minced garlic in a food processor.
- Blend till creamy and smooth.
- Serve alongside whole-grain pita chips, carrot sticks, and cucumber slices.

Nutrition Info:

- Calories: 180
- Carbs: 20g
- Protein: 8g
- Fat: 9g

- Fiber: 6g

Grocery Shopping List:

- Chickpeas (canned or cooked)
- Tahini
- Lemon
- Garlic

Frequent Q&A:

Can I add roasted red peppers for flavor? Yes, it will add a nice smoky touch to the hummus.

Can I use canned hummus instead of making it from scratch? Yes, you can use store-bought hummus if you prefer.

Utensils:

Food processor

17. *Greek Yogurt and Cucumber Dip*

Prep Time: 5 minutes

Serving: 4

Ingredients:

- 1 cup Greek yogurt
- 1/2 cucumber, grated and drained
- 1 clove garlic, minced

- 1 tablespoon fresh dill, chopped

Directions:

- Greek yogurt, grated cucumber, minced garlic, and fresh dill should all be combined in a bowl.
- Stir well to mix.
- Before serving, let the food cool for at least 30 minutes in the refrigerator.
- Serve with sliced bell peppers or whole-grain crackers.

Nutrition Info:

- Calories: 120
- Carbs: 6g
- Protein: 8g
- Fat: 7g
- Fiber: 1g

Grocery Shopping List:

- Greek yogurt
- Cucumber
- Garlic
- Fresh dill

Frequent Q&A:

Can I add lemon juice for extra tanginess? Yes, a splash of lemon juice will enhance the flavors.

Can I use regular yogurt instead of Greek yogurt? Yes, but Greek yogurt has more protein.

Utensils:

Grater for cucumber

Bowl for mixing

18. Mediterranean Stuffed Grape Leaves

Prep Time: 15 minutes

Serving: 6

Ingredients:

- 1 jar grape leaves, drained and rinsed
- 1 cup cooked quinoa or rice
- 1/2 cup chopped fresh parsley
- 1/4 cup chopped fresh mint

Directions:

- Cooked quinoa or rice, parsley, and mint are combined in a dish.
- Place a tiny dollop of the quinoa mixture in the middle of each grape leaf as you go.
- The leaf should be folded in half and rolled up tightly like a cigar.
- Repetition is required with the leftover grape leaves and filling.

- Serve chilled with a squeeze of lemon juice and a sprinkle of olive oil.

Nutrition Info:

- Calories: 150
- Carbs: 30g
- Protein: 4g
- Fat: 1g
- Fiber: 5g

Grocery Shopping List:

- Jar of grape leaves
- Quinoa or rice
- Fresh parsley
- Fresh mint
- Olive oil and lemon juice for serving

Frequent Q&A:

Can I add pine nuts or raisins to the filling? Yes, they will add extra texture and flavor.

Can I make the filling ahead of time? Yes, you can prepare the filling and store it in the refrigerator until ready to use.

Utensils:

Bowl for mixing

19. Mediterranean Tomato Bruschetta

Prep Time: 10 minutes

Serving: 4

Ingredients:

- 2 cups diced ripe tomatoes
- 1/4 cup chopped fresh basil
- 2 cloves garlic, minced
- 2 tablespoons balsamic vinegar

Directions:

- Diced tomatoes, chopped basil, minced garlic, and balsamic vinegar should all be combined in a bowl.
- To enable the flavors to merge, thoroughly combine and set aside for 5 minutes.
- Toast some pieces of whole-grain bread and top them with the tomato bruschetta.

Nutrition Info:

- Calories: 120
- Carbs: 20g
- Protein: 3g
- Fat: 1g
- Fiber: 4g

Grocery Shopping List:

- Ripe tomatoes
- Fresh basil
- Garlic
- Balsamic vinegar
- Whole-grain bread

Frequent Q&A:

Can I add mozzarella cheese on top? Yes, a sprinkle of fresh mozzarella will make it even more delicious.

Can I use white balsamic vinegar? Yes, white balsamic vinegar works well in this recipe too.

Utensils:

Bowl for mixing

20. Mediterranean Stuffed Mushrooms

Prep Time: 15 minutes

Serving: 4

Ingredients:

- 12 large mushrooms
- 1 cup cooked quinoa or couscous
- 1/2 cup chopped sun-dried tomatoes (packed in oil)
- 1/4 cup crumbled feta cheese

Directions:

- Set the oven's temperature to 375°F (190°C).
- The mushroom stems should be cut off and thrown away.
- Combine cooked quinoa or couscous, diced sun-dried tomatoes, and feta cheese in a bowl.
- Insert the quinoa mixture into the caps of each mushroom.
- The stuffed mushrooms should be put on a baking sheet.
- Bake the mushrooms for 15 to 20 minutes, or until they are soft.
- Serve warm.

Nutrition Info:

- Calories: 180
- Carbs: 20g
- Protein: 8g
- Fat: 6g
- Fiber: 3g

Grocery Shopping List:

- Mushrooms
- Quinoa or couscous
- Sun-dried tomatoes (packed in oil)
- Feta cheese

Frequent Q&A:

Can I add spinach to the stuffing? Yes, chopped spinach will add extra nutrients.

Can I use goat cheese instead of feta? Yes, goat cheese is a great alternative.

Utensils:

Baking sheet

Desserts Recipes

21. Mediterranean Fresh Fruit Salad

Prep Time: 10 minutes

Serving: 4

Ingredients:

- 2 cups mixed fruits (grapes, oranges, kiwi, pomegranate seeds)
- 2 tablespoons fresh lemon juice
- 1 tablespoon honey

Directions:

- Fruits should be washed and cut into bite-sized pieces.
- The mixed fruits, fresh lemon juice, and honey should all be combined in a dish.
- Gently toss the fruits until they are evenly covered with the dressing.
- Serve Chilled.

Nutrition Info:

- Calories: 100
- Carbs: 25g
- Protein: 1g
- Fat: 0g
- Fiber: 4g

Grocery Shopping List:

- Grapes
- Oranges
- Kiwi
- Pomegranate seeds
- Fresh lemon
- Honey

Frequent Q&A:

Can I add mint leaves for extra freshness? Absolutely, mint leaves would be a great addition.

Can I use canned fruits? Fresh fruits are recommended for maximum nutritional benefits.

Utensils:

Bowl for mixing

22. Greek Yogurt with Honey and Walnuts

Prep Time: 5 minutes

Serving: 2

Ingredients:

- 1 cup Greek yogurt
- 2 tablespoons honey
- 1/4 cup chopped walnuts

Directions:

- Spoon Greek yogurt into a bowl.
- Yogurt should be covered in honey.
- Add chopped walnuts to the surface.
- Serve right away.

Nutrition Info:

- Calories: 300
- Carbs: 20g
- Protein: 15g
- Fat: 18g
- Fiber: 1g

Grocery Shopping List:

- Greek yogurt
- Honey

- Walnuts

Frequent Q&A:

Can I add cinnamon for extra flavor? Yes, a sprinkle of cinnamon will enhance the taste.

Can I use other nuts? Yes, almonds or pistachios will work well too.

Utensils:

Bowl for serving

23. Mediterranean Orange and Almond Cake

Prep Time: 15 minutes

Baking Time: 30 minutes

Serving: 8

Ingredients:

- 2 large oranges
- 4 eggs
- 1 cup almond flour
- 1/2 cup honey

Directions:

- Set the oven's temperature to 350°F (175°C).

- Oranges should be washed, then cut into quarters with any seeds taken out.
- Oranges should be puréed in a food processor until smooth.
- Beat the eggs and honey together in a separate dish.
- Add the ground almonds and oranges to the egg mixture.
- Combine well after mixing.
- the batter into a cake pan that has been buttered.
- A toothpick placed in the center of the cake should come out clean after baking for 30 minutes.
- Serve the cake once it has cooled.

Nutrition Info:

- Calories: 250
- Carbs: 25g
- Protein: 8g
- Fat: 15g
- Fiber: 3g

Grocery Shopping List:

- Oranges
- Eggs
- Almond flour
- Honey

Frequent Q&A:

Can I use other flours? Yes, you can use a combination of almond flour and regular flour.

Can I add a sprinkle of powdered sugar on top? Yes, it will add a touch of sweetness.

Utensils:

Food processor

Cake pan

24. Mediterranean Yogurt Parfait with Berries and Pistachios

Prep Time: 10 minutes

Serving: 2

Ingredients:

- 1 cup Greek yogurt
- 1/2 cup mixed berries (blueberries, strawberries, raspberries)
- 2 tablespoons chopped pistachios
- 1 tablespoon honey

Directions:

- Greek yogurt, mixed berries, and chopped pistachios should be arranged in a glass.
- On top, drizzle honey.
- Serve right away.

Nutrition Info:

- Calories: 300
- Carbs: 25g
- Protein: 18g
- Fat: 12g
- Fiber: 5g

Grocery Shopping List:

- Greek yogurt
- Mixed berries (fresh or frozen)
- Pistachios
- Honey

Frequent Q&A:

Can I add granola for extra crunch? Yes, granola will add a nice texture.

Can I use other nuts? Yes, almonds or walnuts will work well too.

Utensils:

Glass for serving

25. Mediterranean Chocolate-Dipped Figs

Prep Time: 10 minutes

Serving: 4

Ingredients:

- 8 dried figs
- 1/4 cup dark chocolate chips
- 1 tablespoon chopped pistachios

Directions:

- Use a double boiler or a microwave to melt the dark chocolate chips.
- Each dried fig's bottom half should be dipped into the melted chocolate.
- Put the chocolate-covered figs on a platter that has been covered with parchment paper.
- Top the chocolate with chopped pistachios.
- The chocolate needs ten minutes in the refrigerator to set.
- Serve Chilled.

Nutrition Info:

- Calories: 180
- Carbs: 28g
- Protein: 3g
- Fat: 8g

- Fiber: 5g

Grocery Shopping List:

- Dried figs
- Dark chocolate chips
- Pistachios

Frequent Q&A:

Can I use milk chocolate instead of dark chocolate? Yes, but dark chocolate has more health benefits.

Can I add a pinch of sea salt on top? Yes, it will enhance the flavors.

Utensils:

Microwave or double boiler

Plate lined with parchment paper

Smoothies Recipes

26. Mediterranean Green Smoothie

Prep Time: 5 minutes

Serving: 1

Ingredients:

- 1 cup fresh spinach leaves
- 1/2 cucumber, chopped
- 1/2 green apple, cored and chopped
- 1/2 cup Greek yogurt

Directions:

- Blend fresh spinach, cucumber, green apple, and Greek yogurt together in a blender.
- Blend till creamy and smooth.
- Serve right away.

Nutrition Info:

- Calories: 150
- Carbs: 20g
- Protein: 10g
- Fat: 2g
- Fiber: 5g

Grocery Shopping List:

- Fresh spinach leaves
- Cucumber
- Green apple
- Greek yogurt

Frequent Q&A:

Can I add a splash of almond milk for consistency? Yes, almond milk will make it creamier.

Can I use kale instead of spinach? Yes, kale is a great alternative.

Utensils:

Blender

27. *Mediterranean Berry Smoothie*

Prep Time: 5 minutes

Serving: 1

Ingredients:

- 1 cup mixed berries (blueberries, strawberries, raspberries)
- 1/2 cup Greek yogurt
- 1/2 cup almond milk
- 1 tablespoon honey

Directions:

- Blend the mixed berries, Greek yogurt, almond milk, and honey together in a blender.
- Blend till creamy and smooth.
- Serve right away.

Nutrition Info:

- Calories: 200
- Carbs: 30g

- Protein: 12g
- Fat: 5g
- Fiber: 5g

Grocery Shopping List:

- Mixed berries (fresh or frozen)
- Greek yogurt
- Almond milk
- Honey

Frequent Q&A:

Can I add chia seeds for extra nutrients? Yes, chia seeds will boost the nutritional content.

Can I use soy milk instead of almond milk? Yes, soy milk is a good alternative.

Utensils:

Blender

28. Mediterranean Tropical Smoothie

Prep Time: 5 minutes

Serving: 1

Ingredients:

- 1/2 cup pineapple chunks (fresh or frozen)

- 1/2 cup mango chunks (fresh or frozen)
- 1/2 banana
- 1/2 cup coconut water

Directions:

- Blend the mixed berries, Greek yogurt, almond milk, and honey together in a blender.
- Blend till creamy and smooth.
- Serve right away.

Nutrition Info:

- Calories: 180
- Carbs: 40g
- Protein: 2g
- Fat: 1g
- Fiber: 5g

Grocery Shopping List:

- Pineapple chunks (fresh or frozen)
- Mango chunks (fresh or frozen)
- Banana
- Coconut water

Frequent Q&A:

Can I add a squeeze of lime juice for extra zing? Yes, lime juice will brighten up the flavors.

Can I use pineapple juice instead of coconut water? Yes, pineapple juice will work too.

Utensils:

Blender

29. *Mediterranean Avocado Banana Smoothie*

Prep Time: 5 minutes

Serving: 1

Ingredients:

- 1/2 ripe avocado
- 1 ripe banana
- 1 cup almond milk
- 1 tablespoon honey

Directions:

- The avocado's flesh should be removed and placed in a blender.
- Ripe bananas should be peeled and put in the blender.
- Almond milk should be added, then honey.
- Blend till creamy and smooth.
- Serve right away.

Nutrition Info:

- Calories: 300
- Carbs: 35g
- Protein: 3g
- Fat: 18g
- Fiber: 8g

Grocery Shopping List:

- Avocado
- Ripe banana
- Almond milk
- Honey

Frequent Q&A:

Can I add spinach for extra nutrients? Yes, a handful of spinach will boost the nutritional value.

Can I use cow's milk instead of almond milk? Yes, cow's milk is a good alternative.

Utensils:

Blender

30. Mediterranean Chia Seed Pudding Smoothie

Prep Time: 5 minutes

Serving: 1

Ingredients:

- 2 tablespoons chia seeds
- 1 cup almond milk
- 1/2 teaspoon vanilla extract
- 1/2 cup mixed berries (blueberries, strawberries, raspberries)

Directions:

- Chia seeds, almond milk, and vanilla essence should all be put in a blender.
- Mix the ingredients in a blender on low, then let the mixture aside for five minutes to thicken.
- Blend the mixed berries in the blender until smooth.
- Serve Chilled.

Nutrition Info:

- Calories: 200
- Carbs: 25g
- Protein: 7g
- Fat: 8g
- Fiber: 12g

Grocery Shopping List:

- Chia seeds
- Almond milk
- Vanilla extract
- Mixed berries (fresh or frozen)

Frequent Q&A:

Can I add a drizzle of maple syrup for sweetness? Yes, maple syrup will add a nice touch of sweetness.

Can I use soy milk instead of almond milk? Yes, soy milk is a good alternative.

Utensils:

Blender

Remember to adjust the serving sizes and ingredient quantities according to your specific dietary needs. Enjoy these delicious Mediterranean recipes while managing your high blood pressure with a healthy diet!

CONCLUSION

The Mediterranean diet offers a really all-encompassing and efficient method for accomplishing weight reduction and decreasing high blood pressure. We have looked at the wide range of advantages that come with following this tried-and-true eating strategy, which perfectly balances flavor and health.

With its focus on fresh fruits, vegetables, whole grains, lean meats, and healthy fats, the Mediterranean diet demonstrates to be a sustainable and fun way to lose extra weight and manage hypertension. Its richness of minerals, anti-inflammatory, and antioxidant characteristics not only help with weight reduction but also improve cardiovascular health in general.

This diet's adaptability is one of its main advantages. There will never be a dull time on your culinary journey thanks to the abundance of delectable dishes accessible for breakfast, lunch, supper, snacks, desserts, and smoothies. In addition to preventing diet monotony, this variety also promotes adherence, which makes it simpler to embrace as a long-term lifestyle choice.

Furthermore, people may easily incorporate healthy eating habits into their everyday life thanks to the Mediterranean diet's quick and simple meal preparation alternatives, which fit hectic schedules. Each delicious recipe dispels the myth that eating healthily requires a lot of effort or is monotonous.

Individuals may achieve their weight reduction objectives as well as regulate their high blood pressure by adopting the Delicious Healthy Quick and Easy Mediterranean diet, which lowers the risk of cardiovascular issues. It is clear that this dietary strategy goes beyond passing fads, offering a delightful and supported by science means of achieving better health.

Finally, let's begin on this gastronomic journey and enjoy the tastes of the Mediterranean while nourishing our bodies and savoring the benefits it offers to our health and quality of life. It's important to keep in mind that it's never too late to start making healthier choices, and the Mediterranean diet presents an alluring and gratifying route to a happier, healthier future. Bon appétit!

HAPPY COOKING!